Expressions of my own
' Narcolepsy with Cataplexy '

<u>An onward roller coaster ride, it is...</u>

Solomon A. Briggs

Copyright © 2013 by Solomon Briggs
All rights reserved.

ISBN-13: 978-0989991971
ISBN-10: 0989991970
(Narcoplexic)
Narcoplexic@Narcoplexic.com

Book Note/s:

All of the images, words and/or descriptions within this book are of my own.

Know that, I am not a medical doctor.

However, for years now I have dove deeply within, into grasping and gaining real understanding of this disease. Having read many medical journal entries, articles, research, forums and having had conversations at Mayo Clinic regarding N w/ C; I feel entirely comfortable saying what I say within, in specifics to N w/ or w/out C. Everything within though, is spoken only from my own understanding, along with experience/s relating to living, having Narcolepsy with Cataplexy.

The book size is small, it was the only available option, currently.

Know, this is my first book and I have decided to self-publish it entirely on my own, so please bear with me...

A few common abbreviations that I will use are below:

N = Narcolepsy / C = Cataplexy

N w/ or w/out C = Narcolepsy with or without Cataplexy / PWN = Person/s who has/have Narcolepsy

--For the sketches/drawings within, I've focused exclusively on my own experiences of living, having 'Narcolepsy with Cataplexy.'
All hand drawn using pencils within a 5.5 in. x 8.5 in. recycled sketch paper - book, then minimally graphically edited, by myself.--

Cover:
' Tug of N w/ C War'

There is a tug of war with the brain, a pillow, money and a pill bottle. There are juggling balls falling around me and I'm near the deep restorative sleep (the black, behind me) but never there...

There are 'Four Tetrad Symptoms of Narcolepsy' which are:

Excessive Daytime Sleepiness (E.D.S.) which is the result of being *unable to get 'restorative sleep.'*
PWN *go directly into the REM sleep stage*, when falling asleep, *the sleep pattern is broken*.
To reach the REM sleep stage properly through all sleep stages, it should take approximately 90 minutes.
In the daytime, **PWN** *are sleep deprived and at night,* **PWN** *have disrupted non-restorative sleep*.
Cataplexy is *a minimal loss of muscle tone* (example, *a quick slack or drooping, of the head*) to *'complete temporary muscle paralysis'* (*near instant collapse*), and *is triggered by* most often *'pleasurable emotions'* from *interactions/activity/engagement* but can also be triggered by *anger/anxiety/fear/confrontation/surprise/excitement/exertion* and more (*it is very unpredictable*).
The person is *fully conscious* during an episode / attack, *able to think, hear and* sometimes *see*.
With *'Severe Cataplexy,'* a person will be *entirely paralyzed* and their body will have *zero reflexes*; ragdoll-like.
An episode / attack can be *very brief*, or for others *long*, entirely *depending on each persons own individual case*.
Some, during, *will go into a deep sleep combined with* Sleep Paralysis.
A persons *vitals will appear weak* during an episode / attack, which *is natural* when one is asleep, or paralyzed.
As long as the person *can breathe* during an episode / attack, *there is no danger*; besides perhaps from *during a collapse*.
It is said to be *'an intrusion of REM within the wake state'* as the brain confuses the trigger (*laughter, pleasure, frustration, etc..*) with being a dream. As, when in the REM sleep state, there is a safety measure in place called *'muscle atonia'* (a paralysis of the muscles, or the inability to control one's muscles). Such *is to prevent* one from enacting their dream/s.
Hypnagogic Hallucinations (which I refer to as **Dreams**) tend to *occur close to when falling asleep*, or *close to awakening from sleep*; as they *happen due to the broken stages of sleep*.
You may be somewhat awake and somewhat asleep, *the dream world and the awake world clash, creating some frightening and obscure experiences*; they're very very seemingly real. And, day dreaming is a whole other complexity.
Sleep Paralysis is the *bodies muscle atonia* (*paralyzing*) *not having switched off,* after *exiting* the *REM* sleep stage.
Such tends to *occur right along with* Hypnagogic Dreams, creating all sorts of more fear and/or fright within.
Like Cataplexy, with Sleep Paralysis *you may be stuck in complete temporary paralysis* (able to think, hear and see), although it occurs *when you awaken* rather than being triggered.

Additional Narcolepsy Note/s:

- **N w/ or w/out C**, is a very complex, still very misunderstood and difficult disease.
- The diagnosis is often not made until 10-15 years after the onset of the disease.
- It is said that 1 in every 2,000 people, has **N**.
- Also said is, the impact of **N** in life, *'can be'* comparable to that of the effects in life of living with *M.S. or Parkinsons*.
- Often nearly invisible to others. The condition, the syndrome, the disorder, the disease; is devastatingly real and upfront on the **PWN**. It is broadly difficult and impactful upon the loved ones and/or family of the **PWN**, as well.
- The extent of sleepiness/deprivation which a **PWN w/ or w/out C** experiences, on a regular (often, daily) occurrence, is described as, comparable to not having slept from anywhere between 24, to 72 + hours...
- There are broadly, vast physical and also mental effects upon **PWN w/ or w/out C**. The brain has an excess of Histamines. Along with often many (some more common than others) comorbid conditions and/or diseases.
- **N w/ or w/out C** 'is not' a psychological condition.
- Not every **PWN** actually experiences, all four of the tetrad symptoms; around 70% experience **C**.
- Each **PWN** has a different experience with the disease as a w/hole. Each **PWN** as well, has different degrees of variation/s of each symptom. Some symptom/s will come and go, and change as well; over time.
- There is a genetic susceptibility to developing **N**, and a few certain environmental triggers such as virus (for instance strep-throat, colds, or influenza) and head injury which can increase the susceptibility of developing **N**.
- Comparing the manner of which there is a lack of Insulin, in Diabetics, can be similar (yet vastly different) to how there is a lack of *Orexin* in the brain of **PWN w/ C**; however there is no *Orexin* replacement available..
- There are only symptomatic medications which work for some, but not for all.
- '***Lifestyle Adjustments***' can result in dramatic improvements.
- Naps are a necessity and/or a symptom, more so than a therapy.
- **N** is being considered, an *Auto-Immune Disease*; because within the brain's hypothalamus, *Orexin* has been killed off from an Immune response.
- There is '*No Cure*' for **N w/ or w/out C**, yet...

Note/s About Me:

My name is Solomon Anton Briggs, I am a skateboarder at my core who has a large, and caring heart.

The first year of my life involved serious health matters. At 2 months old I began to have severe seizures.

"Your son appears to be perfectly healthy, besides for the Epileptic seizures;" the doctors told my parents...

After a point, my parents rushed me to Mayo Clinic in Rochester, MN and it was quickly discovered, that I had an excess growth of islets upon my Pancreas; *'Severe Hyperinsulinemia Hypoglycemia.'* At four months old 90-95%+ of my Pancreas was removed and I was very lucky to have survived, and to have been able to live on in the manner which I did, and have, for many years (today I'm in my 30's).

Through childhood I participated in many many activities; *Piano* (state competing), *Soccer* (traveling teams), *Tae-Kwon-Doe* (black belt at age 12), *Spanish* (fluid ~ age 13), *Paper Route/s* (from age 8-16), *Ice Hockey* (traveling J.V. and Varsity), *Percussion* (school band), *Skateboarding* (built two back yard mini-ramps, in high-school)...

Each year, between ages 8 to 21, I spent time living in Nicaragua, in a small village with amazing people that live in a very different manner. When I can manage, I visit them, they are *'Mi Familia, Nica.'* At 18, I drove with 3 friends, a van full of relief aid to the village in Nicaragua, taking 3 weeks being within a *Pastors for Peace Caravan* (for added safety). This was after *Hurricane Mitch* struck them directly, and hard.

The experiences in Nicaragua will always stick with me, having taught me so, so much.

-Throughout my life though, there has been many struggles, difficulties, scares and more. It has been quite a roller coaster ride; yet I do remain strong. Living in a very unusual and quite lonely, at times, dreamland / realm of my own. However, I am so thankful and appreciative of the wonderful Mother that I have who has helped me, continues to, and taught me so much along the way.-

Both *observing and contemplating* are things which I've always done, near endlessly.

Over the past few years I've found writing to be very therapeutic, as *I always have 'a lot' on my mind*.

Recently, I've been *drawing* and *by no means do I have real skills*, I've never given it much time; as was the same for writing, until one day I dove into, doing such.

> Skateboarding could not have helped me adjust to, nor prepared me better for, dealing and living with Cataplexy. <

It has only been a handful of years that I´ve actually known and been diagnosed. Since discovering though, I've come a long way, but it has not been an easy path. Nor were the 28 -30 years prior, not knowing what was causing me, so much grief and also difficulties, throughout just about every element and/or angle within life.

Finally learning what has effected me so much in life, was fascinating in that, it explained so much; my lifelong character traits, behavior/s and mannerism/s are now, with a much more clear and understandable reason…

My parents, can recall that **as an infant** *while tickling me, sometimes I would oddly stop reacting and stare off blankly.*

As a child, *I can recall that my arms would not lift nor respond, while being tickled in the belly, however I could laugh out loud and roll from side to side.*

Around 20 years old, *I began to freeze up and awkwardly have to make my way down to the ground while joking around, laughing, or receiving compliments at home. Such* **over time**, *turned quickly into a brief paralysis, on the ground.*

--**By 28,** *this occurring had* **begun to impact my life in dramatic ways** *and one day I did an internet search of* "*laughter AND paralysis*" *to discover the word:* **Cataplexy.**--

Severe Fatigue and *Migraines* I'd dealt with my entire life. The *tiredness* though *had disguised itself*, *to me*, *but not to others.*

Narcolepsy, at first, seemed so unlikely; yet **Cataplexy** was occuring often, clear, definite and promptly diagnosed.

Through learning and beginning to understand the disease, the symptoms along with so much more, became apparent.

Very much, I want to help spread awareness about this disease. There is no cure and it is life-long.

The fine tuning, trial and error, juggling of *'Lifestyle Adjustments'* **has not been easy and remains to be challenging,** yet it has been '*what has* **brought me much** *of any* relief.'

There is a path, a lifestyle, which works for each one of us.

There is no magical path, nor simple and straight forward one available, within any arms reach.

Learning, recognizing and knowing your own limits, then staying within them, is only one piece of the complex puzzle; as is also, *acceptance and understanding, of the common misunderstanding/s…*

' Normal '

Expressing the seemingly nonexistent 'Normal' which (having Narcolepsy with Cataplexy) is very much a cloudy, gloomy, often rainy-day like; lifestyle.

Day after day; being frequently so, so tired at whatever, random point/s in time.
Near never sleeping well; at least beyond perhaps, a couple of hours.
Awakening tired and as though weights are tied to the body, and you need to sleep, more.
6 - 8 hours of sleep, will feel like 3 hours. But, a headache will develop beyond 8 hours.
-Sigh-
With Cataplexy, fun (and much more) can become restricted and/or a possible danger.
People do just want to have fun, as do I.
Staying within boundaries and limits though, knowing that if you do not, there are and/or will be dangers; takes a dramatic, and invisible, heavy toll upon (any) one.
So much of this is, beyond imagine-able; until you've lived it.
Having so many difficulties with being able to hold and/or fit any job/s, schedule/s, friendship/s, relationship/s, etc…
(¿) 'Normal' somehow (?), it all becomes.

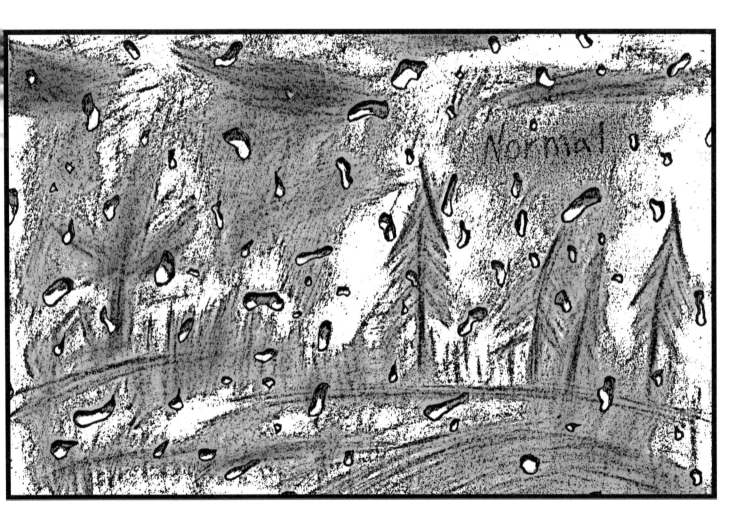

' A-Float-Terrestrial '

That is not supposed to be a smile,
it is a Cataplexy (muscle-less) facial expression.
An element is of feeling as though,
I do not exactly belong on this Planet.
Or, that I am living on an other Planet,
yet am still within this one.
The Moon is only to represent a lonely, and other, Planet.

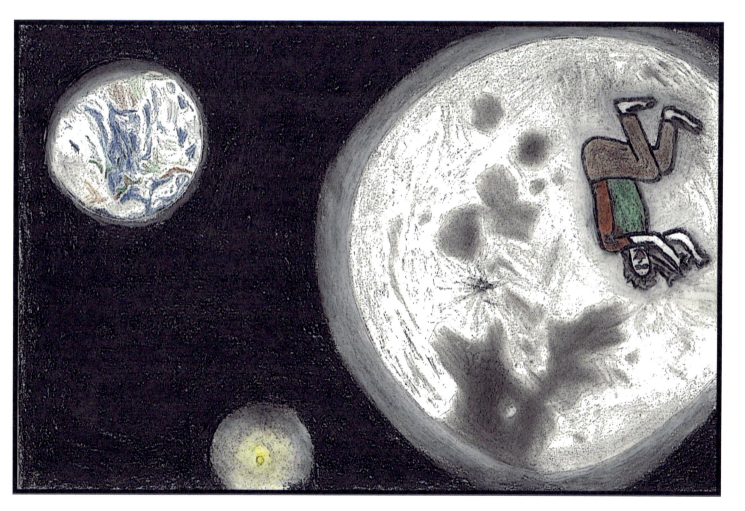

' Acquaintances '

Near never is there any bit of real understanding,
and especially in the beginning,
nor even often beyond it.

Understanding the misunderstanding becomes quite routine.
Though, there is no blame...

' Living A Dream '

Trees and Nature, are what it is all about.
They are also, 'Living A Dream.'
Yet, I can not help but think that many Trees and also places
within Nature (on our Planet today),
don't always have it so well...

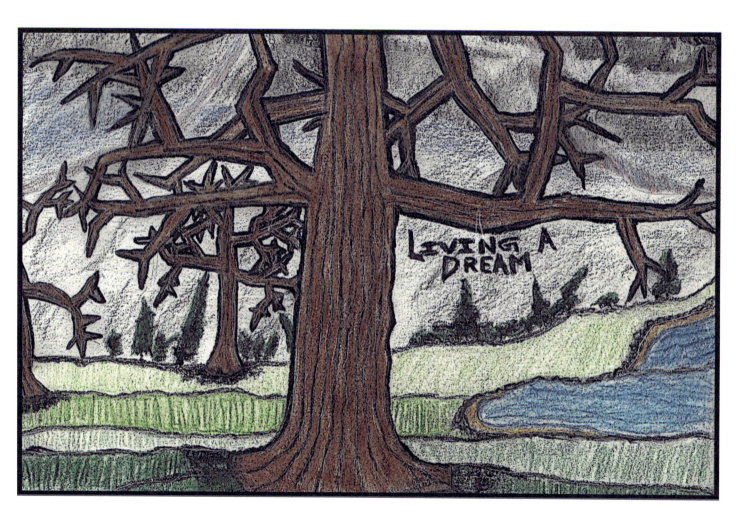

' Endless Dreamz '

An attempt to express the near constant state/s of dreaming.
Be it day, often joyful and night, more so dreadful.

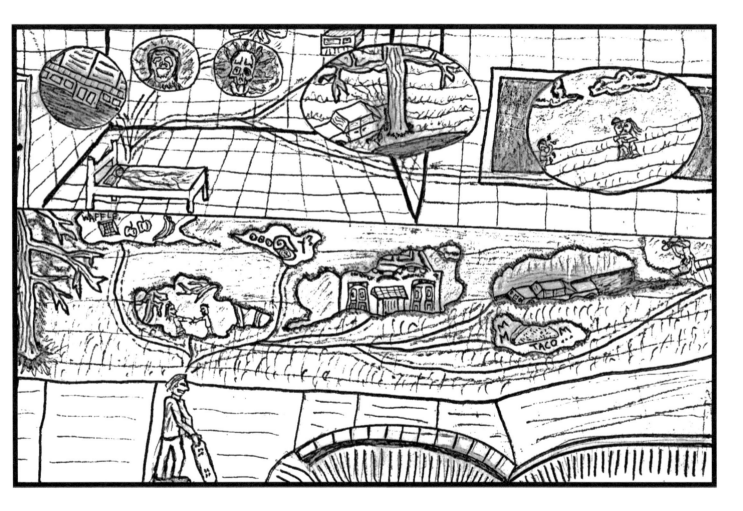

' E'ry Day Coaster '

Dreams occurring day and/or night,
darkness and/or brightness, clear and/or cloudy,
ups and downs, rays and drops,
awake and/or asleep plus somewhere in-between;
with or without vision.

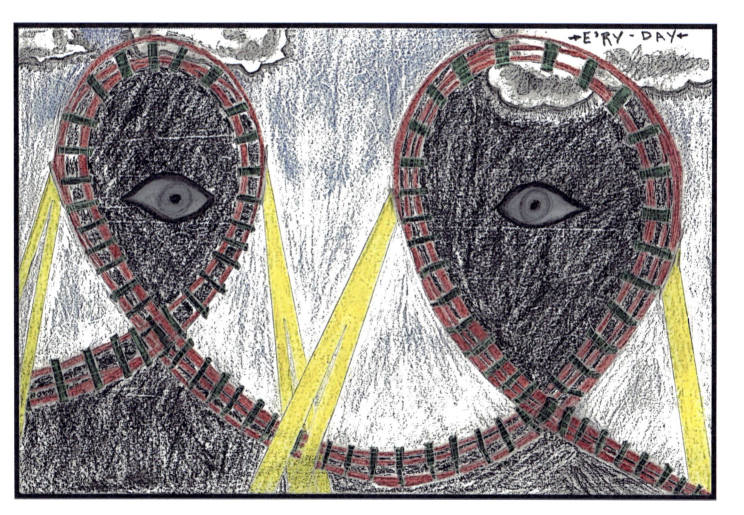

' Life Coaster '

There are the fun moments, the scary moments
and some very uncomfortable moments.
Involving so much; from existing and non-existing relationships, career/s, understanding/s, the (common frequency, pain and difficulties of) comorbidities along with the disease, day to day occurrences, the hoop/s, the twist/s, the speed/s slow to fast, etc…

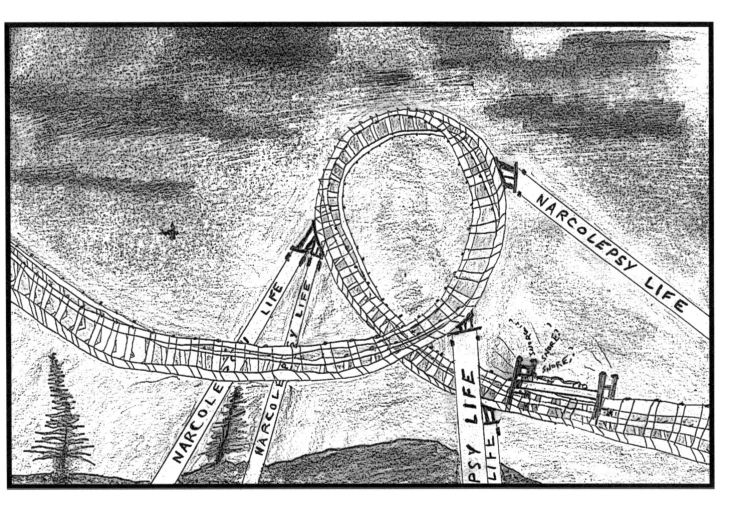

' Bubble Trouble '

A poem going very deep, and into many angles.
Drawn in more of a drop, of some sort.

> This is a bubble, of perhaps my own troubles, yet the fumble is not of mine that crumbles. - The spoken is often broken; annoying and destroying. - Interacting is distracting for some, such causing collapsing. - Annoyed and/or near destroyed, while being tired beyond expired. - Some are numb and some act dumb; strum to become, rather than slum with scum. - Existence is for instance, both dillusions and illusions. - Confusion and intrusion, is often amusion of anothers abussion. - People are equal, yet often distant as though, inexistant. - To care, is a dare, since often others dispair the care as some altered, affair. - Be it one's mistake, or often be it simply that they fake. - Honesty is not policy, nor modesty; today it is simply odyssey. - As today cheats, often result in treats. - Those that lurch in their perch, smirch whatever research. - Dillusions or illusions; confusions do not equal conclusions. - Percieve before you believe, or rather leave before you thieve. - To have perception requires attention, as well as, reflections upon connections. - The result should be affection, of the connections, not rejections of acception. - Assumption is presumption, and results often in corruption. - Being willingly blind is beyond unkind. - Regardless such is heartless. - Dots are to be connected, and perhaps disected. - Knots are to be corrected, as well as then accepted. - Wake up, don't shake up, nor break up. - Be conscious, not obnoxious or blindly unconscious. <

This is a bubbles of perhaps my own troubles; yet the fumble is not of mine that crumbles. The spoken is often broken; annoyed and/or near destroyed, while being tired beyond expired. Some are numb and some act dumb; strum to become annoying. Confusion and intrusion, is often amusion of anothers abusions. People are equal, yet often distant, it simply fake. Honesty is thought rather than some-altered affair. Be it one's mistake, or often be it simply fake. Honesty is thought rather than inexistant, nor research. To have perception requires acceptance as well as rejections; do not. As today cheats, often results in treats. Those that lurch in their perch, search, whatever policy nor modesty. To care becomes a doresire. Today it simply offers attentions confusions as refair. equal conclusions. Perceive before you believe, or rather leave before you think, with scum. Existence is for some, instance, for others, dispersing collapsing illusions and care illusions. -presumption, upon connections. The result should be affection of the connector. Being willing to have perception. Assumption. Regardless, knots are tight, shake up, don't break up. such is heartless. Dots are to be connected, and perhaps dissected, blind is beyond unkind. be corrected, as well as then accepted. Wake up, tis corruption. (break up...

Be conscious, not unconscious.

' Cloud '

*A personal bunch of words.
Trying to hit on what feels like, my own notes,
or what commonly plays on within;
of 'core, day to day (or)deals (the difficulties upon me),
self, and being.'*

NARCOLEPSY WITH CATAPLEXY, SLEEP PARALYSIS, HYPNAGOGIC DREAMS, EXCESSIVE DAYTIME SLEEPINESS, NON-RESTORATIVE SLEEP...

CORE:
CONFIDENCE, AWARENESS, CONTROL, STRENGTH, WILL, INSIGHT, FREQUENCY, RHYTHM, SENSITIVITY, BALANCING, PROPORTIONING, ENHANCING, CONTRASTING, OBSERVING, CONTEMPLATING.

DAY TO DAY DEAL:
JUGGLING, UNDERSTANDING, MISUNDERSTANDING, PRECONCEDED DISMISSALS, JUDGEMENTS, PRESUMPTIONS, SHALLOW INTEREST, MIS-INTERPRETATIONS, ENDLESS MIS-RELATIONS, WEAK CONSIDERATIONS, DISREGARD, DISRESPECT.

SELF:
RECOGNIZING, FIGURING, ACCEPTING, MAINTAINING, CAUTIONING, LIMITING, CONTINUING, CONTAINING, PRESENTING, ACTIVATING, JARRING, SCARRING.

BEING:
CONSCIOUS, OPEN-MINDED, CARING, CONSIDERATE, RESPECTFUL, PASSIONATE, KIND, HUMBLE, HONEST, PROPER, NATURAL, IN-TOUCH, GROUNDED, DRIVEN, OPTIMISTIC, FAIR & EQUAL...

' SmokeN w/ C '

Smoke rising from the flames.

Within the smoke clouds are many personal elements.

One smoke cloud pertains to 'lifestyle' elements to do with,

the difficulties with and/or from, others.

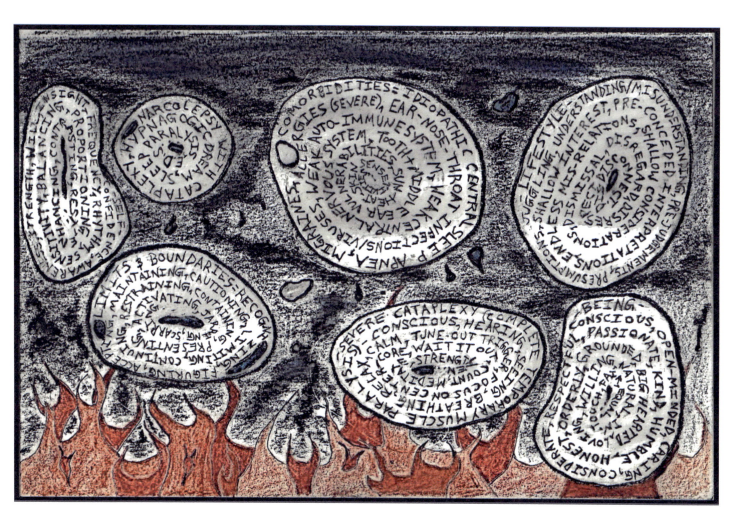

' Live / Think '

We can all choose how we want to Live and Think.
Everything outside of the box has been very good for me.
What lays within the box, has not been good...

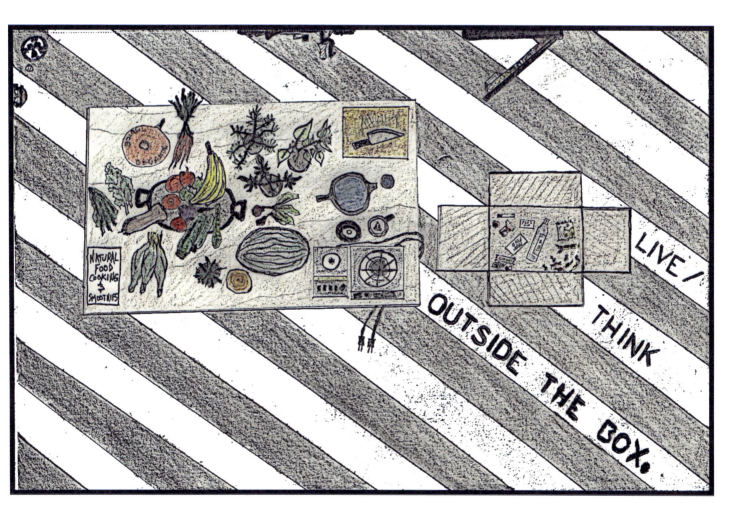

' Box - Void '

A close'r up of the box, within ' Live / Think '.

The point/s and Void within, should be pretty straight forward.

Use -CAUTION- within...

Drinking booze and smoking cigarettes, have never been in my routine.
As for meds, they may be when absolutely necessary and have been in the past,
although for Narcolepsy with Cataplexy they've turned out to
'not have been, more positive than negative.'

-Two important abilities in life, are knowing how to and being able to, both
'agree to disagree'
as well as knowing to and being able to
'respectfully treat others as you would want, or expect, to be treated.'-
> We Are All Equal. <

' Hypnagogic Theater '

The dreams can be so movie like,
that it is as if you are front seat,
or bedside to the film in a private Theater.
A Theater all of your own,
and based most entirely,
upon you.

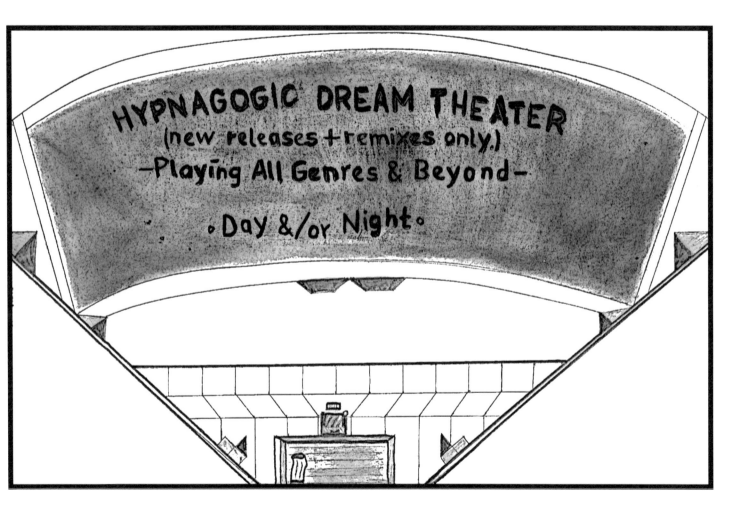

' Hypnagogic Nights '

*Going from one pleasant dream, awakening into another.
One which is near and frightening to you, but then while thinking you've awoken; you find yourself just in an even closer place and within some oddly abstract / cruel / terrifying ordeal.
Often frozen during, unable to react and/or run...
Until that is, after you've finally actually awoken, and are simply in your safe, comfortable (bed) place.
Dreams, within dreams, within deeper dreams, on and on...*

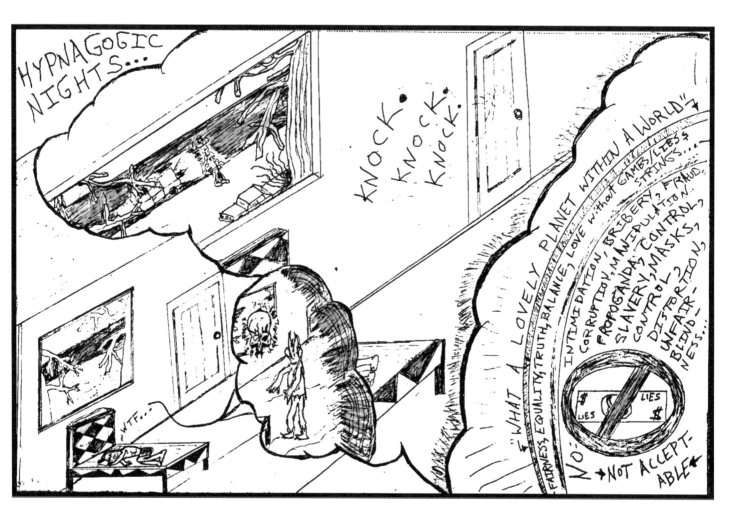

' Day And Night '

Heat and/or cold, difficulty sleeping and/or remaining awake,

frustration/s and/or/with dreams of giant fright/s, all close up...

Be it day-dreaming, be it sight-seeing, be it night-fleeing.

It is to represent the inner hell,

the madness of troubles and struggles;

apart, within, throughout, but most unfortunately all about.

The skull drawn, is influenced by/from an old artist friend
(Thanks, and Much Respect to you, 'Sk8er Jake').

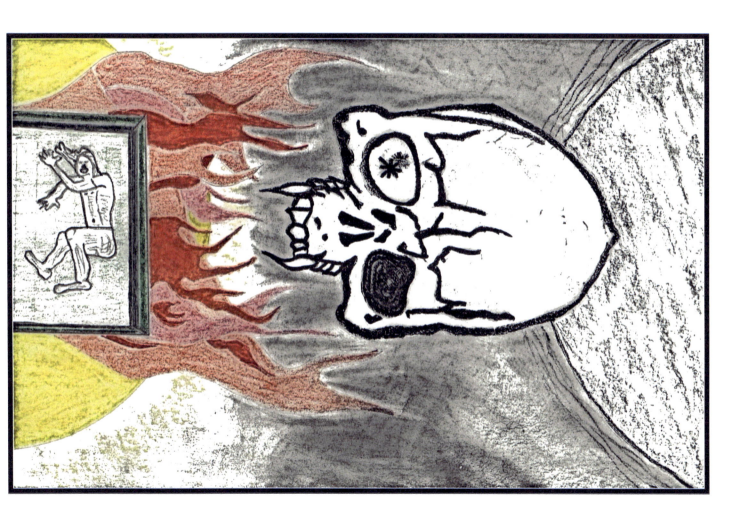

' Ever Sleep '

Dreams can be quite abstract, yet always very real (seemingly). Within both the awake and/or the sleep stage/s, the mind and the physical body gets disrupted, deprived, rattled, disjointed, hindered, distanced, impaired, disadvantaged, obstructed, conducted, missed, dissed (etc...);
it is, has, and can be, of, a tormenting effect/s.
It is hard to stay awake and it is harder to, 'Ever Sleep,' well.

A Note:
Please do not try an relate to being tired, to a PWN w/ or w/out C, such very often is not desired.
Perhaps relate, as to being expired, or fatigued beyond awanting/desire.
Know, that when you can not get what is 'restorative sleep;' 6 hours is not only hard to have in one non-disrupted dose, but upon awakening it feels like 2 to 3 hours of sleep, at most...

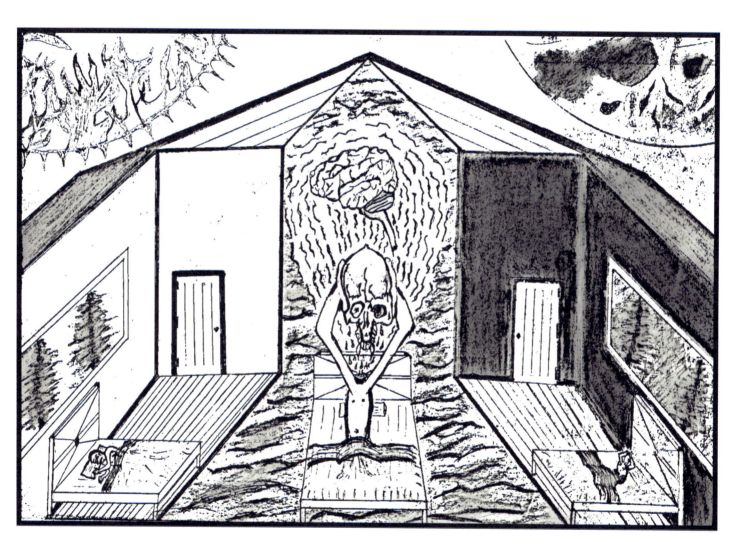

' A Tickle to Paralysis '

My own Cataplexy, at least what I was definitely aware of, as a child. Clueless as to why, thinking somehow that it must just be an aspect of intense laughter.

A Note:

Cataplexy of mental thought, is another even more difficultly abstract, not understood, and nearly invisible aspect of N w/ C; which is just beginning to be recognized by the experts out there...

-- Such is very real. For myself, it has had severe hindering effects upon relationship building, social interaction/s, as well as so much more. --

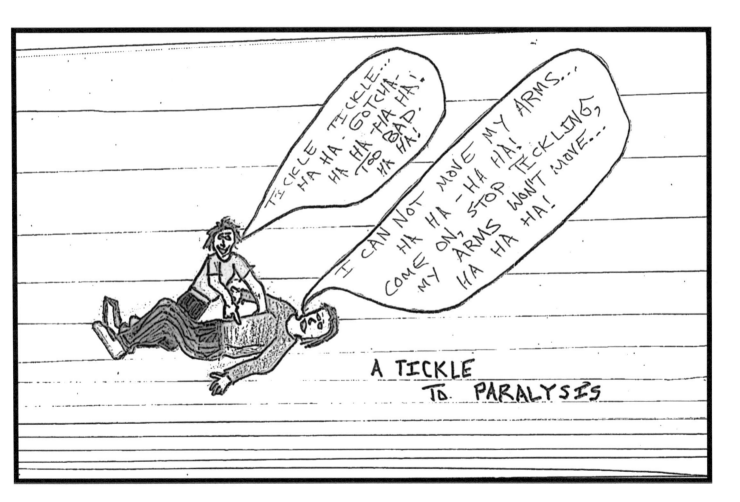

' Severe '

These depict 3, very common, triggers of my own Cataplexy. Watching funny series (for instance, -Curb Your Enthusiasm- by -Larry David-), being asked for change ($) on the street, and being complimented for the food which I've prepared…

A Note:
Living with Cataplexy, one must develop (usually seeming) odd mannerisms of dealing and adjusting to it. There are strange element specifics relating to the 'random triggering'; be it persons (closely known vs. unfamiliar), places (comfortable vs. not), environments (public vs. private), etc…
In my mind, when it comes to Cataplexy the conscious and subconscious are both very much mutually involved, in that one looks out for and attempts to protect the other. Although, remember that I am only speaking from my own experience with it. Skateboarding has taught me such.
In time you can begin to recognize your own boundaries and to know your own limits; yet, there still is no complete/entire predictability, and un/fortunately caution is most always required (safety first).
Think of Swimming. One must always be self-aware, plus of that going on around them, cautious to remain safest; all fronts require attentiveness, yet one can have fun, let-go of-the-focus only-on-caution…

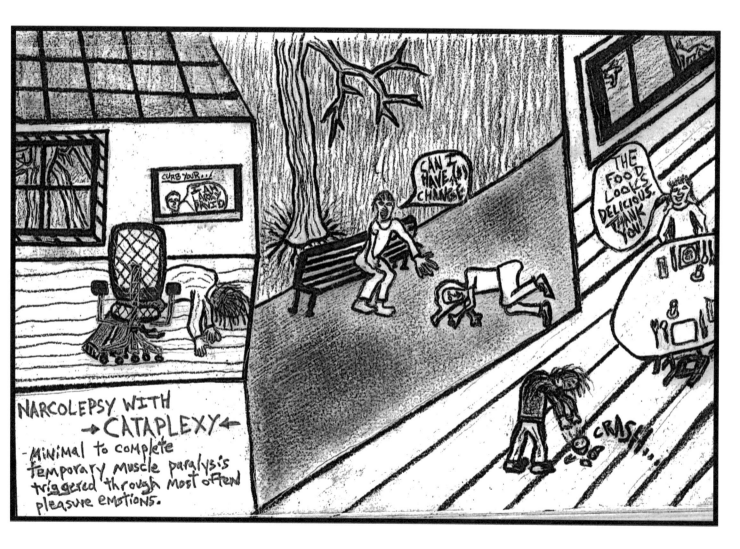

' A. B. C. D. '

A. -being, just a few, possible triggers walking down the street-

B. -Cataplexy triggering; collapse, temporary muscle paralysis-

C. -being what I am thinking to myself, and also what I may be hearing those around me saying-

D. -being some of what those around me say, during and after, the Cataplexy episode-

...You really, can not begin to imagine such...

A tip to others with Cataplexy:

-- Do not fight, nor resist, the Cataplexy.

Calm and Breathe, Focus on Your Core / Center. --

' Cute Zer0 '

A sprawled out Cataplexy occurrence.

Triggered by, Overwhelming kitty Cuteness.

Looks of concern, with Zero Judgements.

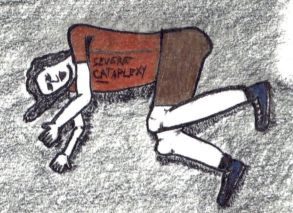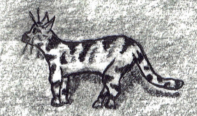

' Hand of Cards '

We each, in life, are dealt a 'Hand of Cards.'
Life is full of vast games, some using different decks.
There are many hands to play, within the games.
Somehow at the grand poker (life-today) game, I seem to have UNO cards.
A good hand perhaps for UNO (!), but definitely not for poker nor for the common, card deck, games.

Personally, I'd not trade my cards, as I do not like poker...
It is, all a trade off.

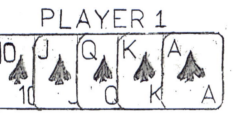
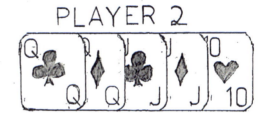
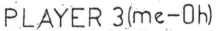
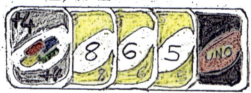
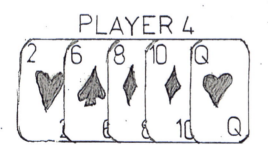
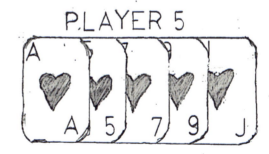

' TwoDay E'ryDay '

The shape is of a skateboard.
The root, is that everyday, is two-day;
as I tend to often end up taking an hour to 3 nap, each day.
And usually that is entirely out of necessity, because if I don't lie
down when the sleep attack hits, I end up asleep in my chair;
which causes my neck to give me a headache.

A Note:
An unfortunate misunderstanding, often, is that PWN
will fall asleep mid-conversation; such has not been ever something
that I personally, have had happen.
That is not to say that it can't or doesn't happen for some, but I don't think it is
so common.

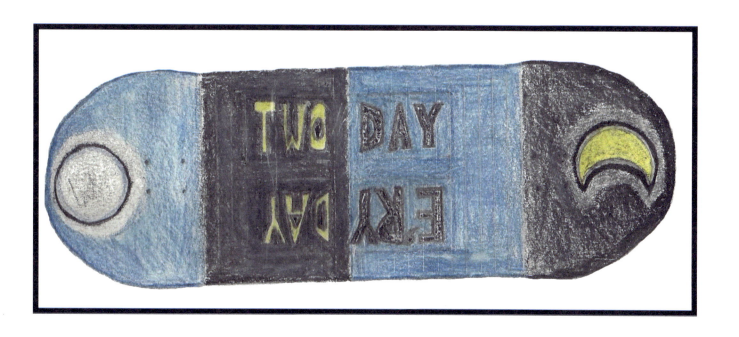

Skateboarding has taught me more about life and living, as well as allowed me to explore; more than any other one thing.

- Rolling is the first step to knowing, on one's way growing. -

' Know '

Very simple, your brain is never awake nor asleep, it simply 'is on.'

One day, it will log off and shut (powering) down.

Something else to know, plus remember:
> We Really ALL, Are, Only ONE. <

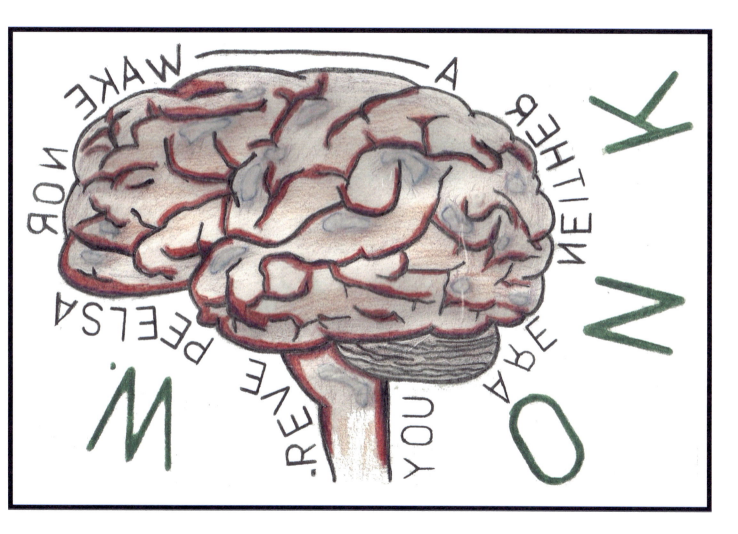

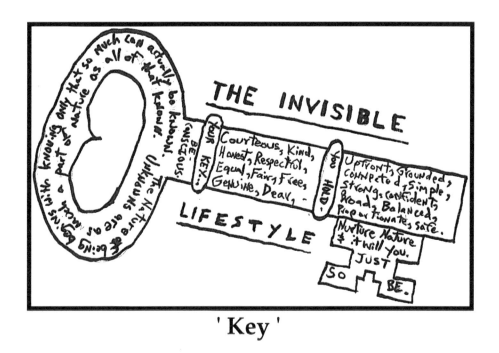

'Key'

What is crucial, in my own eyes, to being a grounded and good, solid person.
- Be conscious.
The nature of being begins with knowing only that so much can actually be known.
Unknowns are as much a part of nature as all of that known.
Nurture Nature & it will you. So Just Be.-

To put the words / labels / diagnosis bluntly, in my own wording / description form:

-'Narcolepsy with Cataplexy' is, becoming considered, an 'Auto-Immune Disease' which directly effects the Brain and the Neurological, Central Nervous and Immune Systems; as well as involving also, the Endocrine System...-

'Narcolepsy' is the inability to get 'restorative sleep' which results in the inability to maintain wakefulness, throughout days and/or nights; so one with it does not sleep well, nor has energy, often.

'Cataplexy' is a symptom of Narcolepsy and is 'a minimal to complete, temporary muscle paralysis,' which is triggered by, most often, pleasurable emotional interactions, engagement, or activity but can be also triggered by many other emotion-tied things.

There is a real need by the general public, as well as by many many doctors, for 'awareness, understanding and recognition' as to what Narcolepsy, along with what Cataplexy, actually is and can be.
Narcolepsy is a condition, a disorder, a syndrome, a disease which is much much more than simply put, a 'sleep disorder.'

- Thank You & Please Be Conscious, Try to Be Understanding of Others, Do Not Be Unconscious... -

' A Skatepark Design '

This, I made (using Rhinoceros 3d Nurbs) right around when my Cataplexy was at its worst ever, collapsing 5-20 times a day (at around 29 years old ~ 2009). During this period of time, a close friend of mine was starting his skatepark construction company, this would have been the first job; but due to numerous complexities, on behalf of the city, it unfortunately never happened.

Also, right around this same time period, I had to turn down a construction job offered, by a friend, in Denmark. After helping (for free) with the design of the bowl, when asked if I wanted to be flown out, sheltered, fed and payed to come help construct, in Denmark; I had to decline. = [

However, I was very glad =] to have helped out my friends and to have had some input on the bowl; which is now built.

Construction and Cataplexy, are not a good mix. And design is too ´cut throat´ (with too much stress along with unknowns) in the skatepark industry.

Everyone wins some, and loses some... On goes the roller coaster ride, which I proudly and thankfully can still say, that I continue (skateboard) rolling on!

(Placed some random skating and construction photos alongside...)

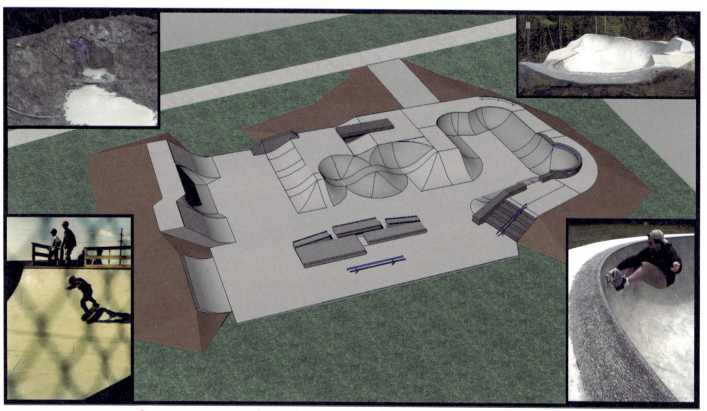

Support your local Skatepark and Skateboarders...

Skateboarding saves lives. The real crime is, not being supportive!

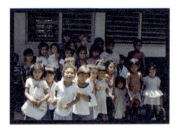
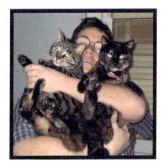
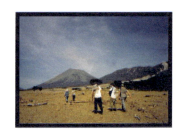

Some random photos...

--**Top left:** Shot in the early 90's in Nicaragua, me with a group of kids.--
--**Top center:** Bronson, Spidita, and I.--
--**Top right:** Anders, John, Maggy, and I; walking the path in Nicaragua of 'Las Casitas' crater, mud slide, after Hurricane Mitch in 1998.--
--**Bottom left:** Small garden from a couple of years back.--
--**Bottom right:** Myself at a Polysomnography (sleep study), 2011.--

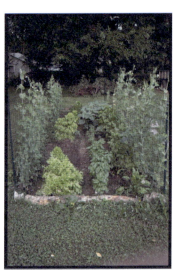
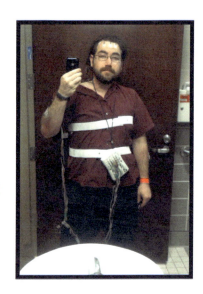

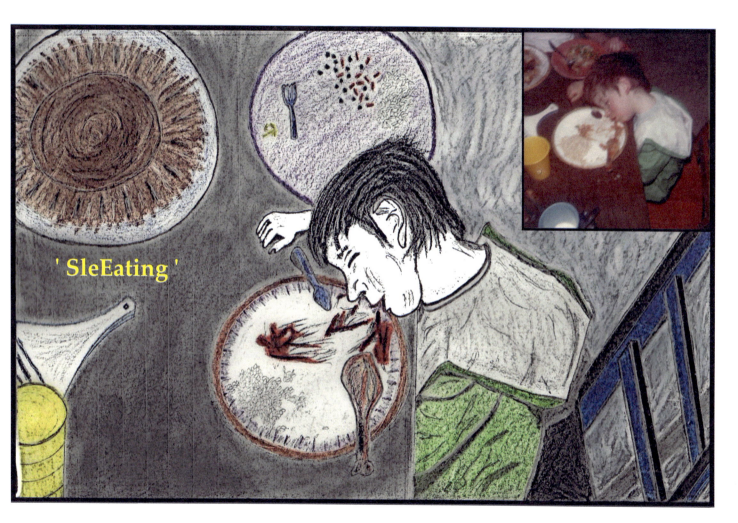

To: Understanding Narcolepsy with or without Cataplexy.

For: All of those who suffer in the dark and/or light,
be it day and/or night.

A Special Thanks To:

1st and Foremost: My Incredible Mother, along with Guillermo (Panson !).

Family: Nate, Russell, Harold (Dad) and Kathleen, Mi Familia Nica -Orbelina, Veronica, Nancy, Tonyo, Felix, y a todos mas-.

Friends: Anders + family, Joel + family, Julian, Bart + the Smiths family, Keddy + family, James + family, Bing + family, Isaac and Ashley, Kava, Nathan + family, Jon + family, JeT, Schulte, Sk8er Jake, Ryan + family, Byron + family, Oliver, Tyson, J.R. + family, Jess, Limpy, Ole, a mis amigos Nicas conocidos, and to the so many more who are out there...
And of course, a shout at my kitties (!); Spidita, Bronson and (R.I.P) Spidey.

(¿) Some of what I may work on, in the future are to do with the following (?):
A memoirs book (possibly a series of them), natural 'Lifestyle Adjustments' which can help PWN w/ or w/out C (specifically, what has helped me), how Skateboarding has related to helping me 'dramatically' with C, Gluten & Dairy Free Cook-book/s, videos regarding N w/ C (there are 2 posted on youtube, already), etc...

[Time Tells!]

Made in the USA
Columbia, SC
05 August 2024